How To Be Vegetarian

Learn How To Be A Vegetarian. Improve Your Lifestyle With These Simple And Flavorful Recipes

Brigitte S. Romeo

How To Be Vegetarian

© Copyright 2021 - All rights reserved.

The content contained within this book may not be reproduced, duplicated or transmitted without direct written permission from the author or the publisher.

Under no circumstances will any blame or legal responsibility be held against the publisher, or author, for any damages, reparation, or monetary loss due to the information contained within this book. Either directly or indirectly.

Legal Notice:

This book is copyright protected. This book is only for personal use. You cannot amend, distribute, sell, use, quote or paraphrase any part, or the content within this book, without the consent of the author or publisher.

Disclaimer Notice:

Please note the information contained within this document is for educational and entertainment purposes only. All effort has been executed to present accurate, up to date, and reliable, complete information. No warranties of any kind are declared or implied. Readers acknowledge that the author is not engaging in the rendering of legal, financial, medical or professional advice. The content within this book has been derived from various sources. Please consult a licensed professional before attempting any techniques outlined in this book.

By reading this document, the reader agrees that under no circumstances is the author responsible for any losses, direct or indirect, which are incurred as a result of the use of information contained within this document, including, but not limited to, errors, omissions, or inaccuracies.

TABLE OF CONTENTS

INTRODUCTION **8**

CHAPTER 1: BREAKFAST RECIPES **12**

1. ONION MILLET 12
2. MANGO-LIME RICE 14
3. BARLEY BREAKFAST BOWL 16
4. PUMPKIN STEEL-CUT OATS 18
5. AMAZING BLUEBERRY SMOOTHIE 20
6. PERFECT BREAKFAST SHAKE 21
7. GO-GREEN SMOOTHIE 22

CHAPTER 2: LUNCH RECIPES **24**

8. BROCCOLI CHEDDAR SOUP 25
9. CREAMY CAULIFLOWER-BROCCOLI SOUP 27
10. CABBAGE AND NOODLES 29

CHAPTER 3: MAIN MEALS RECIPES **30**

11. BAKED ZITI 30
12. BLACK BEAN VEGGIE BURGERS 32
13. TORTILLA PIZZA WITH HUMMUS 34
14. AVOCADO TOAST 36
15. HEMP PORRIDGE WITH PEARS AND BLUEBERRIES 37
16. BASIC BAKED POTATOES 38

CHAPTER 4: VEGETABLES, SALADS AND SIDES RECIPES **40**

17. BUTTERY CORN ON THE COB 40
18. SIMPLY ROASTED ASPARAGUS 43
19. HONEY GLAZED CARROTS 45
20. CREAMY SOUR CREAM MASHED POTATOES 47

21. Mediterranean Spinach Salad ... 49
22. Italian Wedge Salad ... 51
23. Tomato and White Bean Salad ... 53
24. Spicy Cucumber Salad ... 55

CHAPTER 5: DESSERT RECIPES ... 58

25. Blackberry Ice Cream ... 58
26. Chocolate Pudding ... 60
27. Chocolate Brownies ... 61

CHAPTER 6: SNACK RECIPES ... 64

28. Tomato Cream Pasta ... 64
29. Penne Arrabbiata ... 66
30. Hummus Noodle Casserole ... 68
31. Cinnamon Chickpeas ... 70
32. Black-Eyed Peas and Collard Greens ... 72
33. Lentil Bolognese Sauce ... 75
34. Feijoada ... 77

CHAPTER 7: JUICES AND SMOOTHIES RECIPES ... 80

35. Zucchini and Blueberry Smoothie ... 80
36. Tropical Spinach Smoothie ... 82
37. Peach Grapefruit Ginger Smoothie ... 83
38. Great Green Smoothie ... 84
39. Blueberry and Sweet Potato Smoothie ... 85
40. Peanut Butter and Coffee Smoothie ... 86

CHAPTER 8: OTHER RECIPES ... 88

41. Lemony Romaine and Avocado Salad ... 88
42. Strawberry-Coconut Smoothie ... 90
43. Aloha Mango-Pineapple Smoothie ... 91

44.	LENTIL SOUP	92
45.	TRAIL MIX	94
46.	FLAX CRACKERS	95
47.	CRUNCHY GRANOLA	97
48.	CHICKPEA SCRAMBLE BOWL	99
49.	MAPLE FLAVOURED OATMEAL	101
50.	PROTEIN PANCAKES	103

CONCLUSION 106

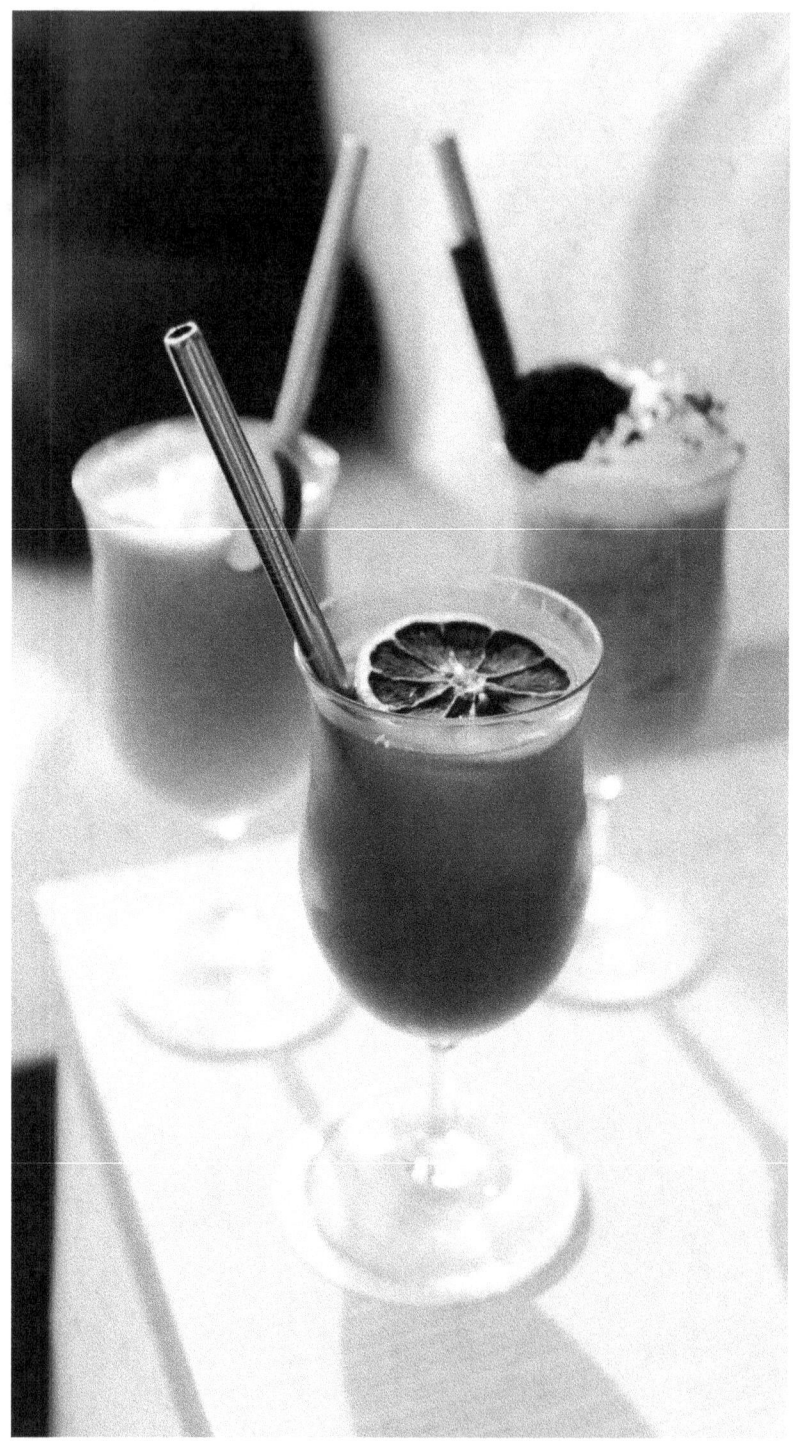

INTRODUCTION

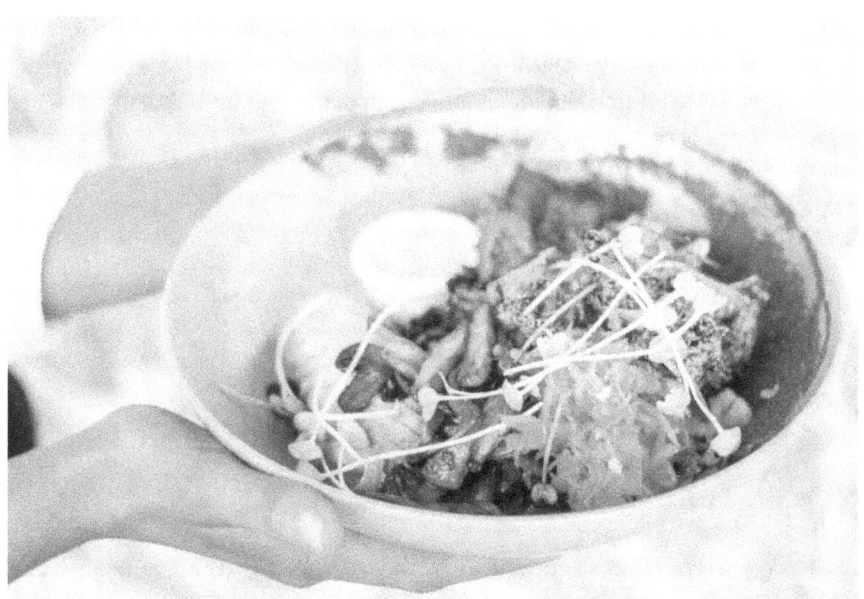

What does it mean to be a vegetarian?

Vegetarian is a person who does not eat meat, poultry, or fish. Vegetarians eat only plant foods such as fruits, vegetables, legumes, and grains or products made from them. Some people think of a vegetarian as a person who does not eat red meat but may consume fish and chicken. Other people consider a vegetarian to be someone who avoids eating all animal flesh, including fish, poultry, and red meat. However, "true" vegetarians avoid the consumption of all meats, including fish and chicken.

So, specifically, what are the foods that one needs to avoid? These are as follows:

- Beef
- Pork

- Lamb

- Veal

- All Game (deer, elk, etc.)

- Any other land mammal that's been fed animal products or by-products such as eggs and dairy (many land mammals are herbivores)

- Fish and Shellfish

- Goose and Duck

- Emu and Alligator

- Any other animal that is not a seafood product

- Animal by-products such as gelatin (e.g., gummy bears)

As a vegetarian, what specific foods do you avoid? For starters, you can limit your consumption of the following:

- Pork and bacon

- Eggs (or eat only eggs that are certified organic or non-cage free)

- Dairy products (or consume only dairy products that are certified organic)

- All products that are made from animals, such as leather shoes, belts, jackets, etc.

What are the substitutes that you use to replace the meat and fish that you avoid?

- Tofu (made from soybeans)

- Tempeh (made from soybeans)

- TVP (textured vegetable protein)

- Seitan (very high in protein, available as steak strips or chicken-style pieces)

- Soy Nuggets/Sausage

Being a vegetarian has its benefits, but there are definitely some challenges as well. If you are considering the option of being a vegetarian, the most important thing to consider is your overall health. However, if you have concerns with the lack of protein in your diet, believe that it's unwise to eat only plant products, or simply crave meat and fish and think you can't give them up without feeling hungry or deprived, then the choice of becoming a vegetarian may not be the right one for you.

This vegetarian cookbook will help you get a delicious and healthy recipe on the table that will make your life less stressful. A good recipe doesn't need a long list of ingredients to make it tasty, and while preparing meals may seem hard. You can eat together a healthy family food in the same amount of time you'd need to order takeout!

This vegetarian cookbook will show you a variety of dishes you can make with easy-to-find ingredients. This is the perfect practical guide for anyone looking to make a variety of delicious meals that are healthy. It includes recipes for breakfast, lunch, dinner, appetizers, and desserts, as well as those for snacks and sides. Whether looking to lose weight or just eat more healthily, this cookbook will make it easier than ever before!

So, let us begin the journey.

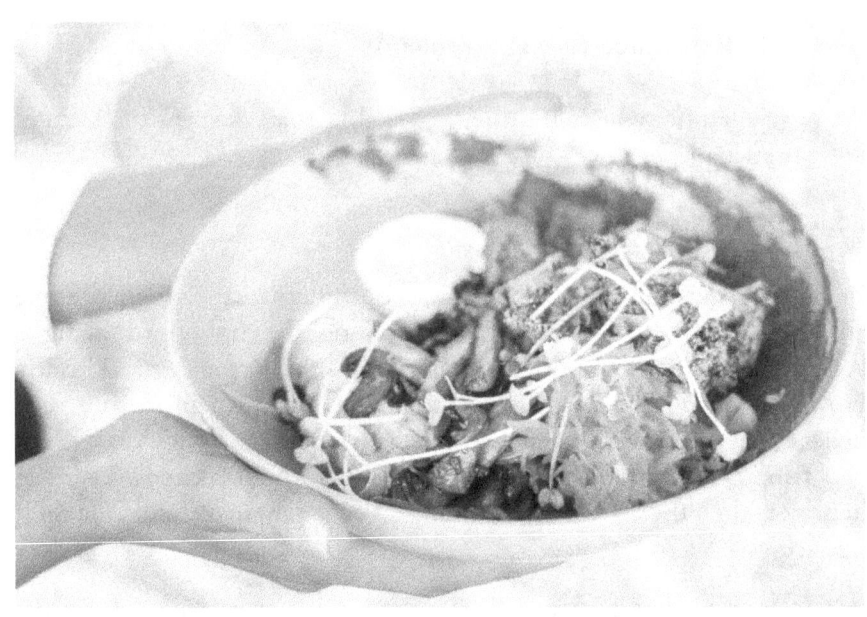
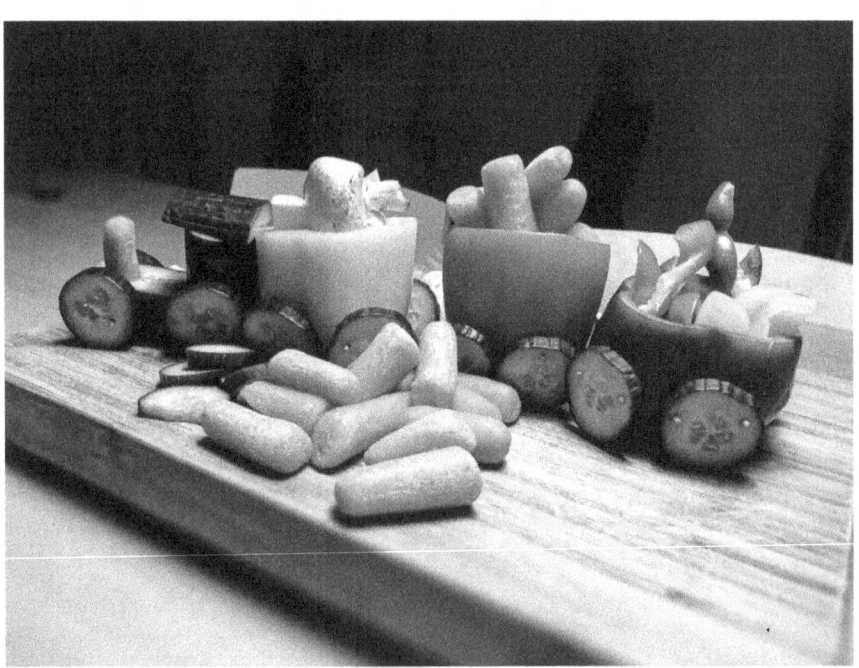

CHAPTER 1:

BREAKFAST RECIPES

1. Onion Millet

Preparation Time: 5 minutes

Cooking Time: 20 minutes

Servings: 2

Ingredients:

- ½ tablespoon vegetable oil
- 1 red onion, chopped
- ½ cup millet
- ½ teaspoon ground black pepper
- 1 cup vegetable broth

Directions:

1. Heat the oil in an Instant Pot on Sauté mode. Stir in the onion, and cook until almost tender. Stir in millet and continue cooking until coated with oil. When the onion is tender, and millet begins to brown lightly, season with pepper, and pour in the vegetable broth. Close Instant Pot with the pressure valve to Sealing. Cook on Manual for 10 minutes followed by 10-minute natural pressure release.
2. Open Instant Pot.
3. Enjoy.

Nutrition: Calories 262 Fat 6.3g Cholesterol 0mg Carbohydrate 42.4g Fiber 5.6g

2. Mango-Lime Rice

Preparation Time: 5 minutes

Cooking Time: 10 minutes

Servings: 2

Ingredients:

- ½ cup brown rice
- 1 cup water
- ¼ tablespoon fresh lime juice
- 1/8 cup chopped fresh rosemary
- ¼ mango, peeled, pitted, and cut into 1/2 inch cubes

Directions:

1. Combine water, brown rice, and lime juice, mango in an Instant Pot.
2. Close the pressure-release valve. Select Manual and set the pot at High Pressure for 10 minutes. At the end of the cooking time, allow the pot to sit undisturbed for 10 minutes, then release any remaining pressure.

3. Serve with fresh rosemary.

4. Enjoy.

Nutrition: Calories 210 Fat 2g Cholesterol 0mg Carbohydrate 45.2g Fiber 3.9g

3. Barley Breakfast Bowl

Preparation Time: 5 minutes

Cooking Time: 30 minutes

Servings: 6

Ingredients:

- 1½ cups pearl barley
- 3¼ cups water
- Large pinch salt
- 1½ cups dried cranberries or cherries
- 3 cups sweetened vanilla plant-based milk
- 2 tablespoons slivered almonds (optional)

Directions:

1. In a large saucepan over high heat, combine the barley, water, and salt. Bring to a boil. Cover the pot, reduce the heat to low, and simmer for 25 to 30 minutes, stirring occasionally, until the water is absorbed.

2. Divide the barley into 6 jars or single-serving storage containers. Add ¼ cup of dried cranberries to each. Pour ½ cup of plant-based milk into each. Add 1 teaspoon of slivered almonds (if using) to each. Close the jars tightly with lids.

Nutrition: Calories 249 Fat 2g Cholesterol 0mg Carbohydrate 54g Fiber 9g

4. **Pumpkin Steel-Cut Oats**

Preparation Time: 2 minutes

Cooking Time: 35 minutes

Servings: 4

Ingredients:

- 3 cups water
- 1 cup steel-cut oats
- ½ cup canned pumpkin purée
- ¼ cup pumpkin seeds (pepitas)
- 2 tablespoons maple syrup
- Pinch salt

Directions:

1. In a large saucepan, bring the water to a boil.
2. Add the oats, stir, and reduce the heat to low. Simmer until the oats are soft, 20 to 30 minutes, continuing to stir occasionally.

3. Stir in the pumpkin purée and continue cooking on low for 3 to 5 minutes longer. Stir in the pumpkin seeds and maple syrup, and season with the salt.

4. Divide the oatmeal into 4 single-serving containers. Let cool before sealing the lids.

Nutrition: Calories 121 Fat 5g Carbohydrate 17g Fiber 2g

5. **Amazing Blueberry Smoothie**

Preparation Time: 5 minutes

Cooking Time: 0 minutes

Servings: 1

Ingredients:

- ½ avocado
- 1 cup of frozen blueberries
- 1 cup of raw spinach
- Pinch of sea salt
- 1 cup of soy or unsweetened almond milk
- 1 frozen banana

Directions:

1. Blend everything in a powerful blender until you have a smooth, creamy shake.
2. Enjoy your healthy shake and start your morning on a fresh note!

Nutrition: Fat 9 g Carbohydrates 32 g Protein 5 g Calories: 220

6. Perfect Breakfast Shake

Preparation Time: 5 minutes

Cooking Time: 0 minutes

Servings: 1

Ingredients:

- 3 tablespoons of raw cacao powder
- 1 cup of soy/almond milk
- 2 frozen bananas
- 3 tablespoons of natural peanut butter

Directions:

1. Use a powerful blender to combine all the ingredients.
2. Process everything until you have a smooth shake.
3. Enjoy a hearty shake to kick start your day.

Nutrition: Calories: 330 Fat 15 g Carbohydrates 41 g Protein 11 g

7. Go-Green Smoothie

Preparation Time: 5 minutes

Cooking Time: 0 minutes

Servings: 1

Ingredients:

- 2 tablespoons of natural cashew butter
- 1 ripe frozen banana
- 2/3 cup of unsweetened coconut, soy, or almond milk
- 1 large handful of kale or spinach

Directions:

1. Put everything inside a powerful blender.
2. Blend until you have a smooth, creamy shake.
3. Enjoy your special green smoothie.

Nutrition: Calories: 390 Fat19 g Carbohydrates 42 g Protein15 g

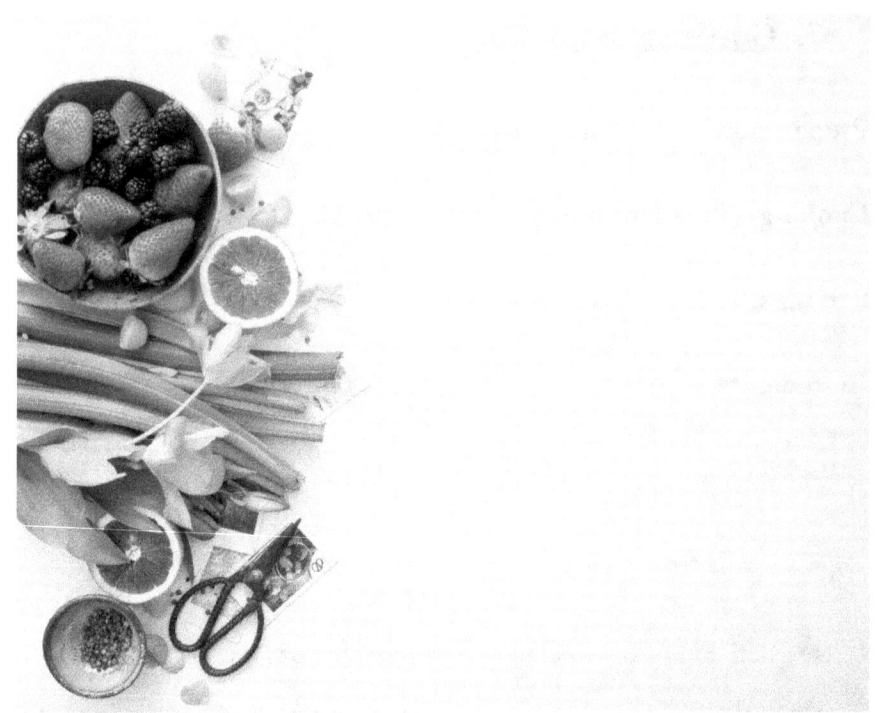

CHAPTER 2:

LUNCH RECIPES

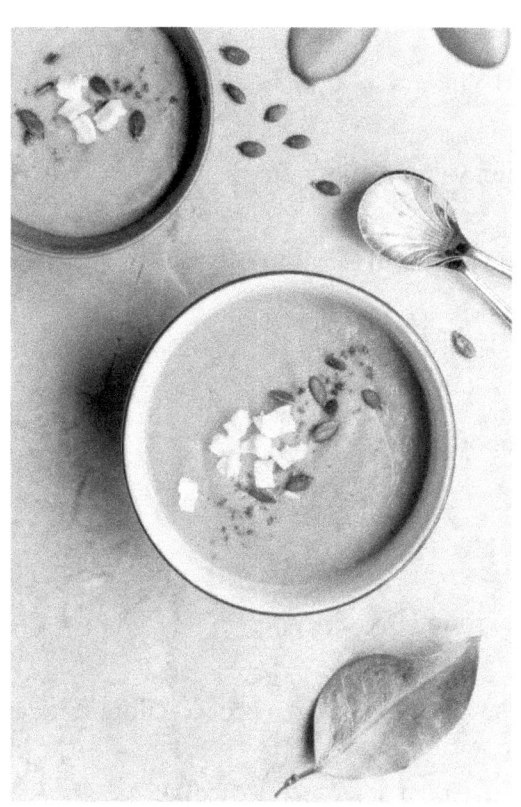

8. Broccoli Cheddar Soup

Preparation Time: 10 minutes

Cooking Time: 8 hours

Servings: 5

Ingredients:

- 2 cups vegetable broth
- 1 pound Yukon Gold potatoes, peeled
- 1 medium yellow onion, diced
- 2 scallions, minced
- 1 teaspoon garlic powder
- ¼ teaspoon ground thyme
- Salt
- Freshly ground black pepper
- 1 (1-pound) package frozen broccoli florets, thawed and drained
- ½ cup shredded extra-sharp Cheddar cheese
- ½ cup milk

- 1 tablespoon unsalted butter

Directions:

1. Combine the broth, potatoes, onion, scallions, garlic powder, and thyme in the slow cooker. Season with salt and pepper.

2. Cover and wait for it to cook on low for 8 hours.

3. Carefully transfer the contents of the slow cooker to a blender in batches if necessary. Purée until smooth, making sure to vent the blender lid for steam. Add three-quarters of the broccoli. Pulse three or four times. Then wait to get the consistency of the soup that you desired.

4. Pour the soup back into the slow cooker. Add the Cheddar, milk, butter, and remaining broccoli and stir. Season with salt and pepper, if needed.

5. Cook until warmed through. Serve.

Nutrition: Calories: 194 Total Fat: 8g Cholesterol: 20mg Sodium: 431mg Total Carbohydrates: 24g Fiber: 5g Protein: 10g

9. Creamy Cauliflower-Broccoli Soup

Preparation Time: 10 minutes

Cooking Time: 8 hours

Servings: 6

Ingredients:

- 2 pounds cauliflower florets
- 2 scallions, minced
- 2 cups vegetable broth
- 1 teaspoon onion powder
- 1 teaspoon garlic powder
- ¼ teaspoon dried thyme
- ½ teaspoon salt, plus more for seasoning
- ¼ teaspoon ground black pepper
- 1 (12-ounce) package frozen broccoli florets
- ½ cup grated Parmesan cheese
- ¼ cup heavy cream

Directions:

1. Combine the cauliflower, scallions, broth, onion powder, garlic powder, thyme, salt, and pepper in a slow cooker.

2. Cover and wait for it to cook on low for 8 hours.

3. Carefully transfer the contents of the slow cooker to a blender in batches if necessary. Purée until smooth, making sure to vent the blender lid for steam. Pour the puréed soup back into the slow cooker.

4. Stir in the broccoli, Parmesan cheese, and cream. Cover and set it on high for 10 minutes, or until heated through.

5. Season with salt and pepper, if needed. Serve soup into bowls and then garnish with more Parmesan cheese, if desired.

Directions: Calories: 124 Total Fat: 5g Cholesterol: 14mg Sodium: 642mg Carbohydrates: 14g Fiber: 6g Protein: 10g

10. Cabbage and Noodles

Preparation Time: 5 minutes Cooking Time: 5 minutes

Servings: 2

Ingredients:

- 1 cup wide egg noodles
- 1 1/2 tablespoon butter
- 1 small onion
- 1/2 head green cabbage, shredded
- Salt and pepper to taste

Directions:

1. Add egg noodles, butter, water, onion, green cabbage, pepper, and salt to Instant Pot. Place lid on Instant Pot and lock into place to seal. Pressure Cook on High Pressure for 4 minutes. Use Quick Pressure Release.
2. Serve and enjoy.

Nutrition: Calories 183 Fat 6.8g Cholesterol 31mg Carbohydrate 27.2g Fiber 5.9g

CHAPTER 3:

MAIN MEALS RECIPES

11. Baked Ziti

Preparation Time: 15 minutes

Cooking Time: 20 minutes

Servings: 6

Ingredients:

- 16 oz. vegan ziti pasta
- 15 oz. canned chickpeas
- 2 cups baby spinach
- 4 cups tomato sauce
- 1 ½ cup non-dairy cheese

Directions:

1. Preheat the oven to 400 F.

2. Cook the ziti pasta base on packaging instruction. Strain the pasta and return the pasta to the pot.

3. Add the chickpeas, spinach, and tomato sauce to the pasta and mix well. Pour half the pasta mixture into your oven dish and spread equally. Sprinkle with ¾ cup sugar. Layer the rest of the pasta mixture on top and sprinkle with the remaining cheese.

4. Cover the dish with aluminum foil and bake for 20 minutes.

5. Serve while still warm.

Nutrition: Calories: 405 Carbs: 53g Fat: 11g Protein: 25g

12. Black Bean Veggie Burgers

Preparation Time: 10 minutes

Cooking Time: 20 minutes

Servings: 4

Ingredients:

- 30 oz. canned, drained black beans
- ¾ cup rolled oats
- 1 canned chipotle pepper in adobo chili sauce, as well as 1 tbsp. of the sauce
- 1 avocado
- Olive oil for cooking

Directions:

1. Preheat your oven to 350 F.
2. Rinse your beans and place them on your baking tray. Bake for 10 minutes until the beans become dry to the touch and start to split.

3. Place the beans in your food processor along with the oats, chipotle pepper, and sauce. Pulse until the ingredients start to stick together. This should take roughly 20 seconds.

4. Mash the avocado in a bowl and add the bean mixture. Stir and fold together until everything forms a dough-like ball. Form the mixture into four balls and flatten them into patties.

5. Heat some olive oil in a frying pan over medium heat. Fry the patties for 3 - 4 minutes on each side.

6. Serve the patties on some whole grain, vegan buns together with all your favorite burger toppings.

Nutrition: Calories: 112 Carbs: 21g Fat: 0g Protein: 7g

13. Tortilla Pizza with Hummus

Preparation Time: 10 minutes

Cooking Time: 17 minutes

Servings: 1

Ingredients:

- 1 - 2 vegan tortilla shells (depending on how hungry you are)
- ⅓ cup hummus per tortilla shell
- Toppings of your choice
- ½ - ¾ cup grated vegan mozzarella per tortilla shell
- Chopped thyme

Directions:

1. Preheat the oven to 400 F.
2. Place the tortilla shells on your baking tray and bake for 7 minutes until golden brown. Remove from the oven and let cool while preparing your toppings. Do not turn off your oven.

3. Spread the hummus over the tortilla shells and add your toppings. Cover with the vegan mozzarella. Sprinkle with a little chopped thyme.

4. Put back into the oven and bake for 10 minutes.

5. Slice the pizza shell and serve immediately.

Nutrition: Calories: 214 Carbs: 16g Fat: 14g Protein: 12g

14. <u>Avocado Toast</u>

Preparation Time: 5 minutes

Cooking Time: 0 minutes

Servings: 1

Ingredients:

- Salt, one quarter teaspoon
- Black pepper, one half teaspoon
- Avocado, one peeled and sliced thinly
- Whole grain bread, two slices toasted

Directions:

1. Slice the avocado while the bread is toasting. Lay the slices of avocado onto the toast and sprinkle on the pepper and salt.

Nutrition: Calories: 362 Carbs: 30g Fat: 25g Protein: 10g

15. Hemp Porridge with Pears And Blueberries

Preparation Time: 5 minutes

Cooking Time: 5 minutes

Servings: 1

Ingredients:

- Almond milk, one cup
- Blueberries, one half cup
- Hemp seeds, one half tablespoons
- Pear, one medium-sized sliced
- Porridge oats, one half cup

Directions:

1. In a medium-sized saucepan over a medium heat, pour in the porridge and the almond milk. Bring the mix to a boil and then turn down the heat and let the porridge simmer for five minutes. Spoon the porridge into a bowl and top it with the blueberries, hemp seeds, and pears and serve.

Nutrition: Calories: 463 Carbs: 78g Fat: 11g Protein: 17g

16. Basic Baked Potatoes

Preparation Time: 5 minutes

Cooking Time: 60 minutes

Servings: 5

Ingredients:

- 5 medium Russet potatoes or a variety of potatoes, washed and patted dry
- 1 to 2 tablespoons extra-virgin olive oil or aquafaba
- ¼ teaspoon salt
- ¼ teaspoon freshly ground black pepper

Directions:

1. Preheat the oven to 400°F.
2. Pierce each potato several times with a fork or a knife. Brush the olive oil over the potatoes, then rub each with a pinch of the salt and a pinch of the pepper. Place the potatoes on a baking sheet and bake for 50 to 60 minutes until tender.

3. Place the potatoes on a baking rack and cool completely. Transfer to an airtight container or 5 single-serving containers. Let cool before sealing the lids.

Nutrition: Calories: 171 Carbs: 34g Fat: 3g Protein: 4g

CHAPTER 4:

VEGETABLES, SALADS AND SIDES RECIPES

17. Buttery Corn on the Cob

Preparation Time: 15 minutes

Cooking Time: 15 minutes

Servings: 6

Ingredients:

- 6 large ears of corn, shucked

- 1 cup whole milk

- 3 tablespoons butter, melted

- Salt

- Black pepper

Directions:

1. Fill a large pot halfway with water. Bring to a boil over medium-high heat.

2. Add the corn (the cobs can be cut in half if you want) and milk. Turn heat to medium and then cook the corn for 6 to 10 minutes, depending on how tender you like it, with a few more minutes if you like it more tender.

3. Turn the heat off, but you can keep the corn warm in the pot for up to an hour until you're ready to serve it.

4. Remove corn from the water and drizzle the butter over it. Season with salt and pepper to taste.

5. Technique Tutorial: Here is the easiest way to shuck corn. Cut off the stalk end of each cob right above the first row of kernels with a sharp knife. Place 3 ears of corn on a microwave-safe plate. Microwave for about 60 seconds. Hold the corn by the uncut end in one hand while shaking the ear up and down until

the cob slips free, leaving the husk and silk behind. Repeat the other 3 ears of corn.

Nutrition: Calories: 160 Carbs: 36g Fat: 3g Protein: 6g

18. Simply Roasted Asparagus

Preparation Time: 5 minutes

Cooking Time: 20 minutes

Servings: 6

Ingredients:

- 2 pounds asparagus, trimmed
- 2 tablespoons olive oil
- 1 teaspoon garlic powder
- ½ teaspoon salt
- ¼ teaspoon black pepper

Directions:

1. Preheat the oven to 400°F.
2. In a large bowl, put the asparagus with olive oil and sprinkle with garlic powder, salt, and pepper. Make sure to coat well. Place on a large rimmed baking sheet.
3. Roast it for 15 minutes or until the asparagus is as tender as you like it.

4. Ingredient Tip: Pick bunches of asparagus that have a rich green color and purple highlights with a small amount of white on the bottom. Stalks must be firm, and the tips should not be mushy. To trim the asparagus, just snap off the bottoms as the perfect amount of the stalk will snap right off. It is best not to store asparagus for more than a few days and to cook it as soon as possible.

Nutrition: Calories: 76 Carbs: 12g Fat: 2g Protein: 6g

19. Honey Glazed Carrots

Preparation Time: 5 minutes

Cooking Time: 25 minutes

Servings: 6

Ingredients:

- 1 pound carrots, peeled
- ½ teaspoon salt
- 2 teaspoons dried parsley
- 2 tablespoons butter, melted
- 2 tablespoons honey

Directions:

1. Preheat oven to 425F, then prepare a rimmed baking sheet with parchment paper.
2. Cut the carrots into 2-inch-thick rounds.
3. In a medium bowl, mix salt, parsley, butter, and honey until evenly coated. Spread the carrots on the baking sheet.
4. Bake carrots 20 to 25 minutes or until tender.

5. Easy Variation: Substitute a 1-pound bag of baby carrots for regular carrots. Then you can skip the peeling and cutting.

Nutrition: Calories: 80 Carbs: 13g Fat: 2g Protein: 0g

20. Creamy Sour Cream Mashed Potatoes

Preparation Time: 5 minutes

Cooking Time: 25 minutes

Servings: 6

Ingredients:

- 3 pounds potatoes, cubbed in 2 inches
- 3 tablespoons butter, plus more if desired
- ¾ cup milk
- ¾ cup sour cream
- 1 teaspoon salt and black pepper

Directions:

1. Place potatoes with water in a pot on medium-high heat. Bring to a boil and reduce the heat to low. Cover and simmer the potatoes for 15 to 20 minutes or until they are tender. Drain the potatoes in a colander and return them to the pot.

2. Add the butter, milk, sour cream, salt, and pepper to the potatoes. Mash it until smooth. Add a little more milk if necessary.

3. Serve topped with an additional pat of butter, if desired.

4. Technique Tutorial: To mash potatoes, use a masher in an up-and-down motion, and keep mashing until you get the desired consistency. Use a wooden spoon to blend them together after they have been mashed. If you would like extra-creamy potatoes, you can mash the potatoes, then beat them with a hand beater for about 60 seconds or until they are the smoother texture you desire.

Nutrition: Calories: 110 Carbs: 10g Fat: 3g Protein: 3g

21. Mediterranean Spinach Salad

Preparation Time: 10 minutes

Cooking Time: 0 minutes

Servings: 6

Ingredients:

- 10 to 12 ounces baby spinach
- 1 cup canned chickpeas, rinsed and drained
- ½ cup crumbled feta cheese
- 2 cups grape tomatoes
- ⅓ cup Simple Italian Vinaigrette or your favorite bottled vinaigrette

Directions:

1. In a large bowl, mix the spinach, chickpeas, cheese, and tomatoes.
2. Toss the salad with the dressing right before serving.
3. Prep Tip: Baby spinach is sold in 6-ounce bags and 10-ounce bags. Use either two smaller bags or one larger bag. You can

usually find bags of prewashed spinach that is ready to add to your salad.

Nutrition: Calories: 548 Carbs: 57g Fat: 27g Protein: 21g

22. Italian Wedge Salad

Preparation Time: 10 minutes

Cooking Time: 0 minutes

Servings: 4

Ingredients:

- ½ head iceberg lettuce
- 1 cup grape tomatoes, halved
- 6 ounces diced salami
- 6 ounces diced provolone cheese
- ⅓ cup Simple Italian Vinaigrette or your favorite bottled vinaigrette
- Optional: ½ cup sliced black olives

Directions:

1. Cut the lettuce into 4 equal wedges. Place in an individual plates or on a large platter.
2. Top each lettuce wedge with evenly divided amounts of tomatoes, salami, and cheese. Drizzle the dressing on the salads.

3. Top with black olives, if desired.

4. Prep Tip: Buy the salami and provolone cheese from the deli section at your grocery store. You can get it thickly sliced, then just dice it up before tossing it in the salad.

Nutrition: Calories: 200 Carbs: 2g Fat: 10g Protein: 0g

23. Tomato and White Bean Salad

Preparation Time: 10 minutes

Cooking Time: 0 minutes

Servings: 6

Ingredients:

- 1 can white beans
- 1 pint grape tomatoes, halved
- 3 tablespoons chopped fresh basil
- ⅓ Cup crumbled feta cheese
- ¼ cup Simple Italian Vinaigrette or your favorite bottled vinaigrette
- Black pepper

Directions:

1. In a bowl, mix the beans, tomatoes, basil, and cheese.
2. Drizzle the dressing over the salad and mix well.
3. Add pepper to taste.

4. Leftovers: Store leftovers overnight in an airtight container in the refrigerator. This salad is great served on a bed of greens for lunch the next day.

Nutrition: Calories: 220 Carbs: 41g Fat: 1g Protein: 15g

24. Spicy Cucumber Salad

Preparation Time: 10 minutes

Cooking Time: 0 minutes

Servings: 4

Ingredients:

- 2 tablespoons rice vinegar
- 1 teaspoon sea salt
- 1 tablespoon sugar
- 1 tablespoon sesame oil
- 1 large English cucumber, ends trimmed, thinly sliced
- Pinch red pepper flakes

Directions:

1. Mix the rice vinegar, salt, sugar, and sesame oil until the sugar dissolves in a bowl.
2. Add the cucumber slices and red pepper to the bowl. Mix and season with more salt, if desired.
3. Refrigerated before serving.

4. Ingredient Tip: English cucumbers are large, seedless cucumbers found in the produce section of the grocery store. You can substitute 3 smaller pickling (kirby) cucumbers, if you can't find English cucumbers.

Nutrition: Calories: 60 Carbs: 5g Fat: 3g Protein: 4g

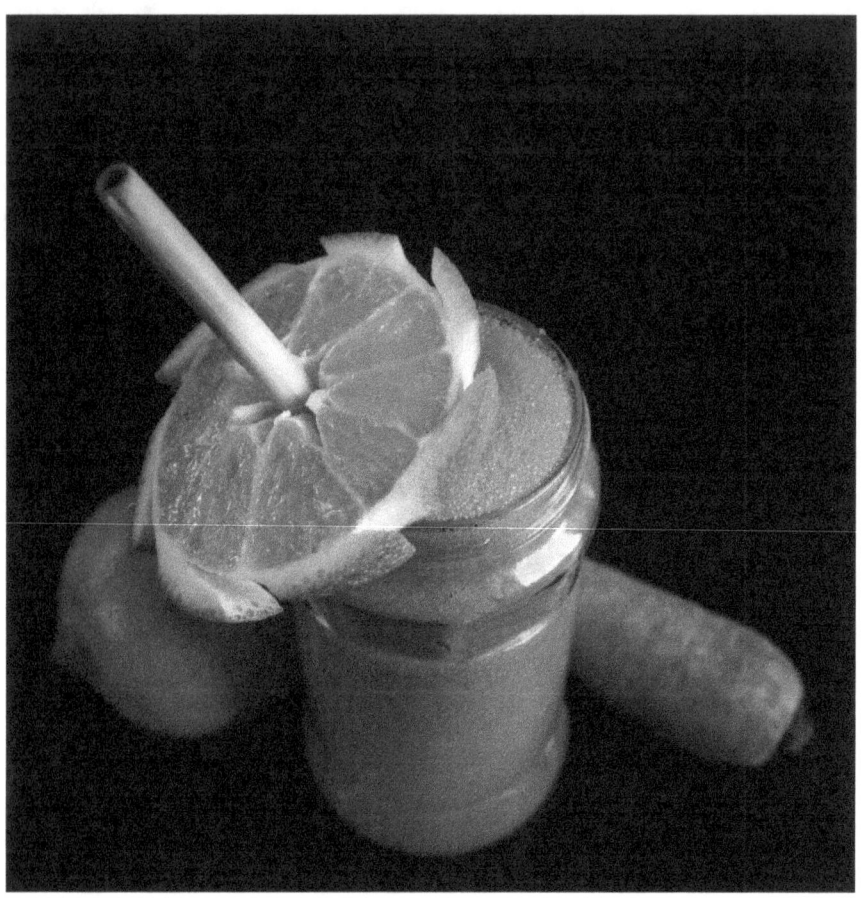

CHAPTER 5:

DESSERT RECIPES

25. Blackberry Ice Cream

Preparation Time: 5 minutes

Cooking Time: 0 minutes

Servings: 1

Ingredients:

- 1 ½ peeled and frozen banana
- 1 cup frozen blackberries
- 1 tbsp. plant-based protein powder
- Fresh mint leaves
- Ice cubes

Directions:

1. In your food processor, blend the frozen berries and banana until it starts to form a single mass.

2. Add the mint leaves and protein powder. Add one or two ice cubes and pulse to help the ingredients blend better.

3. Serve immediately.

Nutrition: Calories: 210 Total fat: 19g Carbohydrates: 13g Protein: 2g

26. Chocolate Pudding

Preparation Time: 5 minutes

Cooking Time: 0 minutes

Servings: 2

Ingredients:

- 1 avocado
- 1 ripe banana
- 4 tbsp. cocoa powder
- 2 tbsps. Dark maple syrup

Directions:

1. Blend the avocado, banana, cocoa powder, and maple syrup in your food processor until everything is thoroughly blended.
2. Chill at least for 30 minutes in the fridge before serving.

Nutrition: Calories: 110 Total fat: 23g Carbohydrates: 2g Protein: 0g

27. Chocolate Brownies

Preparation Time: 5 minutes

Cooking Time: 25 minutes

Servings: 12

Ingredients:

- 2 bananas
- ½ cup cashew butter
- ¼ cup dark maple syrup
- ¼ cup cocoa powder
- 1 ½ tbsp. plant-based, vanilla-flavored protein powder

Directions:

1. Preheat the oven to 350 F.
2. Mash the bananas with a fork in a bowl. Add the cashew butter, maple syrup, cocoa powder, and mix well until a batter forms.
3. Put batter into the dish and bake for 20 - 25 minutes, according to your preferences. Turn around after the first 15 minutes.

4. Let the brownies cool down before cutting them into squares. Enjoy and serve!

Nutrition: Calories: 223 Total fat: 21g Carbohydrates: 15g Protein: 3g

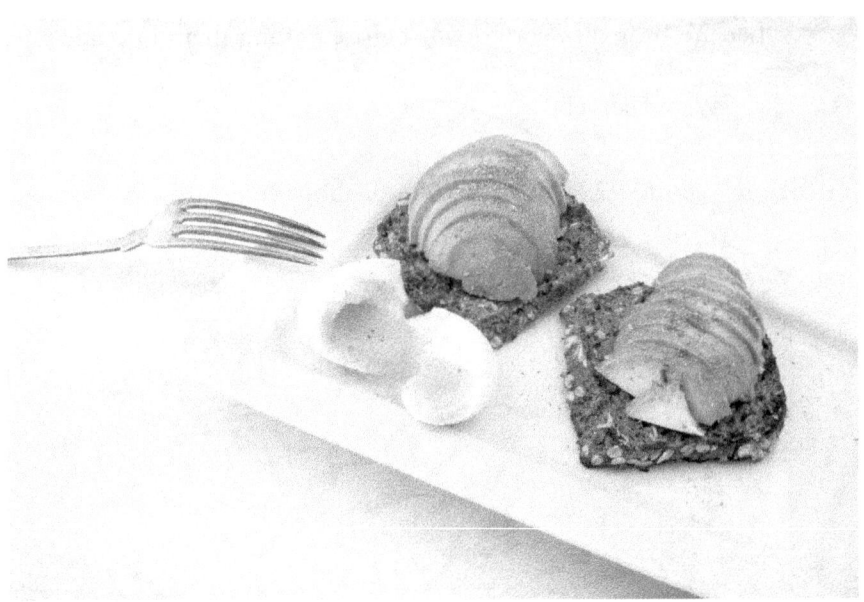

CHAPTER 6:

SNACK RECIPES

28. Tomato Cream Pasta

Preparation Time: 5 minutes

Cooking Time: 10 minutes

Servings: 4

Ingredients:

- 1 (28-ounce) can crushed tomatoes
- 1 tablespoon dried basil
- ½ teaspoon garlic powder
- 10 ounces penne, rotini, or fusilli (about 3 cups)
- ½ teaspoon salt, plus more as needed
- 1½ cups water or unsalted vegetable broth

- 1 cup unsweetened nondairy milk or creamer

- 2 cups chopped fresh spinach (optional)

- Freshly ground black pepper

Directions:

1. Using a pressure cooker, combine the tomatoes, basil, garlic powder, pasta, salt, and water.

2. Close then lock the lid. Ensure that it is safe, then select high pressure. After, set it for 4 minutes.

3. Once done, release the pressure slowly for 5 minutes. Then release any remaining pressure. Make sure to do some extra precautionary when using a pressure cooker.

4. Once done and the pressure is released, remove the lid carefully. Stir in the milk and spinach (if using). Taste and season with more salt, if needed, and pepper.

5. On your pressure cooker, select Sauté or Simmer. Cook until sauce thickens for 4 to 5 minutes and the greens wilt.

Nutrition: Calories: 321 Total fat: 3g Protein: 14g Sodium: 365mg Fiber: 9g

29. Penne Arrabbiata

Preparation Time: 10 minutes

Cooking Time: 20 minutes

Servings: 4

Ingredients:

- 1 red onion, diced
- 2 garlic cloves, minced
- 1 teaspoon olive oil
- 1 (28-ounce) can crushed tomatoes
- 1½ cups water
- 10 ounces penne pasta (about 3 cups)
- ½ to 1 teaspoon red pepper flakes
- ½ teaspoon salt, plus more as needed
- Freshly ground black pepper

Directions:

1. On your electric pressure cooker, select Sauté. Add the red onion, garlic, and olive oil. Cook for 4 to 5 minutes and stir occasionally, until the onion is softened.

2. Add the tomatoes, water, pasta, red pepper flakes, and salt. Cancel Sauté.

3. Close then lock the lid. Ensure that it is safe, then select high pressure. After, set it for 4 minutes.

4. Once done, release the pressure slowly for 5 minutes. Then release any remaining pressure. Make sure to do some extra precautionary when using a pressure cooker.

5. Once done and the pressure is released, remove the lid carefully. Add salt and black pepper if needed.

Nutrition: Calories: 327 Total fat: 3g Protein: 14g Sodium: 317mg Fiber: 9g

30. Hummus Noodle Casserole

Preparation Time: 5 minutes

Cooking Time: 15 minutes

Servings: 4

Ingredients:

- 1 cup hummus
- 3¼ to 3½ cups water and/or unsalted vegetable broth
- 10 ounces penne, bow tie, or small shell pasta (about 3 cups)
- 3 or 4 celery stalks, chopped
- ½ teaspoon sweet paprika
- ½ teaspoon dried thyme
- 1 cup peas
- ¼ to ½ cup fresh parsley, finely chopped
- Salt
- Freshly ground black pepper

Directions:

1. Using a pressure cooker, stir together the hummus and water until mostly combined. Add the pasta, celery, paprika, and thyme. If you like your peas fully cooked, add them here, as well as the parsley if you want it to merge into the sauce.

2. Close then lock the lid. Ensure that it is safe, then select high pressure. After, set it for 4 minutes.

3. Once done, release the pressure slowly for 5 minutes. Then release any remaining pressure. Make sure to do some extra precautionary when using a pressure cooker.

4. Once done and the pressure is released, remove the lid carefully. Stir in the peas and parsley. Season with salt and pepper if desired.

Nutrition: Calories: 434 Total fat: 10g Protein: 16g Sodium: 30mg Fiber: 11g Fat: 7g

31. Cinnamon Chickpeas

Preparation Time: 8 minutes

Cooking Time: 42 minutes

Servings: 4 to 6

Ingredients:

- 1 cup dried chickpeas
- 2 cups water
- 2 teaspoons ground cinnamon, plus more as needed
- ½ teaspoon ground nutmeg (optional)
- 1 tablespoon coconut oil
- 2 to 4 tablespoons unrefined sugar or brown sugar, plus more as needed

Directions:

1. Soak chickpeas overnight and drain. Rinse the chickpeas, then put them in your electric pressure cooker's cooking pot.

2. Add the water, cinnamon, and nutmeg (if using). Then lock the lid. Ensure that it is safe, then select high pressure. After, set it for 30 minutes.

3. Once done, release the pressure slowly for 15 minutes. Then release any remaining pressure. Make sure to do some extra precautionary when using a pressure cooker.

4. Once pressure is released, carefully remove the lid. Drain any excess water from the chickpeas and add them back to the pot.

5. Stir in the coconut oil and sugar. Taste and add more cinnamon, if desired. Select Sauté and cook for about 5 minutes, stirring the chickpeas occasionally, until there's no liquid left and the sugar has melted onto the chickpeas. Transfer into a bowl, then toss it with additional sugar if you want to add a crunchy texture.

Nutrition: Calories: 253 Total fat: 7g Protein: 11g Sodium: 9mg Fiber: 10g

32. Black-Eyed Peas and Collard Greens

Preparation Time: 5 minutes

Cooking Time: 50 minutes

Servings: 4 to 6

Ingredients:

- 1 yellow onion, diced
- 1 tablespoon olive oil
- 1 cup dried black-eyed peas
- 2 cups water or unsalted vegetable broth
- ¼ cup chopped sun-dried tomatoes
- ¼ cup tomato paste or natural ketchup
- 1 teaspoon smoked paprika
- Pinch red pepper flakes (optional)
- 4 large collard green leaves
- Salt
- Freshly ground black pepper

Directions:

1. On your electric pressure cooker, select Sauté. Add the onion and olive oil and cook for 3 to 4 minutes, stirring occasionally, until the onion is softened. Add the black-eyed peas, water, tomatoes, tomato paste, paprika, and red pepper flakes (if using) and stir to combine. Cancel Sauté.

2. Close then lock the lid. Ensure that it is safe, then select high pressure. After, set it for 30 minutes.

3. Once done, release the pressure slowly for 15 minutes. Then release any remaining pressure. Make sure to do some extra precautionary when using a pressure cooker.

4. Trim off the thick parts of the collard green stems, then slice the leaves lengthwise in half or quarters. Roll them up together, then finely slice them into ribbons. Sprinkle the sliced collard greens with a pinch of salt and massage it into them with your hands to soften.

5. Once pressure is released, carefully unlock and remove the lid. Add the collard greens and ½ teaspoon of salt to the pot, stirring to combine and letting the greens wilt in the heat. Taste and

season with salt and pepper. If you want your greens cooked more, select Sauté again for another few minutes.

Nutrition: Calories: 267 Total fat: 5g Protein: 15g Sodium: 332mg Fiber: 13g

33. Lentil Bolognese Sauce

Preparation Time: 10 minutes

Cooking Time: 40 minutes

Servings: 3

Ingredients:

- 12 ounces mushrooms, sliced (about 4½ cups)
- 1 onion, diced
- 1 tablespoon olive oil or vegan margarine
- ½ cup dry white wine or red wine
- 2 cups dried green lentils
- 1 (28-ounce) can crushed tomatoes
- 2 cups water or unsalted vegetable broth
- ¼ to ½ teaspoon salt
- Freshly ground black pepper

Directions:

1. On your electric pressure cooker, select Sauté. Add the mushrooms, onion, and olive oil and toss to combine. Cover the pot but do not lock the lid, and cook for 7 to 8 minutes, until the onion and mushrooms are slightly browned. Add wine, then cook again for 1 to 2 minutes until wine is evaporated.

2. Stir in the lentils, tomatoes, and water. Cancel Sauté.

3. Close then lock the lid. Ensure that it is safe, then select high pressure. After, set it for 10 minutes.

4. Once done, release the pressure slowly for 20 minutes. Then release any remaining pressure. Make sure to do some extra precautionary when using a pressure cooker.

5. Once released and pressure is out, carefully remove the lid. Use salt and pepper to taste.

Nutrition: Calories: 303 Total fat: 4g Protein: 19g Sodium: 114mg Fiber: 21g

34. Feijoada

Preparation Time: 10 minutes

Cooking Time: 1 hour and 5 minutes

Servings: 6 to 8

Ingredients:

- 1 large onion, diced
- 3 or 4 garlic cloves, minced
- 1 tablespoon olive oil
- 2 cups dried black beans
- 4 cups water and/or unsalted vegetable broth
- 1 tablespoon ground cumin
- 1 tablespoon smoked paprika
- 1 tablespoon dried oregano
- Salt
- ¼ cup fresh cilantro, chopped

Directions:

1. On your electric pressure cooker, select Sauté. Add the onion, garlic, and olive oil. Cook for 5 minutes and stir until the onion is softened. Add the black beans, water, cumin, paprika, and oregano, stirring to combine. Cancel Sauté.

2. Close then lock the lid. Ensure that it is safe, then select high pressure. After, set it for 30 minutes.

3. Once done, release the pressure slowly for 30 minutes. Then release any remaining pressure. Make sure to do some extra precautionary when using a pressure cooker.

4. Once pressure is released, carefully remove the lid. Taste and season with ½ to 1 teaspoon of salt. If your beans are not quite soft enough, or if you have too much liquid, select Sauté or Simmer and cook, uncovered, for 10 to 15 minutes more. Stir in the cilantro just before serving.

5. Serve with rice, sautéed collard greens or kale, and orange wedges. For an authentic cultural experience, toast ½ cup cassava flour in 2 to 3 tablespoons coconut oil in a small skillet,

then put it in medium heat for 3 to 5 minutes until browned; sprinkle over the finished dish.

Nutrition: Calories: 268 Total fat: 4g Protein: 16g Sodium: 199mg Fiber: 16g

CHAPTER 7:

JUICES AND SMOOTHIES RECIPES

35. Zucchini and Blueberry Smoothie

Preparation Time: 3 minutes

Cooking Time: 0 minutes

Servings: 2

Ingredients:

- 1 cup frozen blueberries
- 1 cup unsweetened almond milk
- 1 banana
- 1 zucchini, peeled and chopped

Directions:

1. Combine all ingredients in a high-speed blender and blend until smooth.

Nutrition: Calories: 244 Carbohydrates: 19g Total fat: 4g Protein: 20g

36. Tropical Spinach Smoothie

Preparation Time: 3 minutes

Cooking Time: 0 minutes

Servings: 2

Ingredients:

- 1/2 cup crushed ice or 3-4 ice cubes
- 1 cup coconut milk
- 1 mango, peeled and diced
- 1 cup fresh spinach leaves
- 4-5 dates, pitted
- 1/2 tsp. vanilla extract

Directions:

1. Combine all ingredients in a high-speed blender and blend until smooth.

Nutrition: Calories: 130 Carbohydrates: 26g Total fat: 0g Protein: 1g

37. Peach Grapefruit Ginger Smoothie

Preparation Time: 5 minutes

Cooking Time: 0 minutes

Servings: 2

Ingredients:

- ½ frozen banana
- 1 teaspoon of fresh mint, chopped
- 1 cup frozen peaches
- 1 teaspoon ground ginger
- 1 cup grapefruit juice

Directions:

1. Blend well in the blender, slowly at first, and then increasing the speed to break down the fruit and blend it well.

Nutrition: Calories: 187 Carbohydrates: 32g Total fat: 2g Protein: 13g

38. Great Green Smoothie

Preparation Time: 5 minutes

Cooking Time: 0 minutes

Servings: 4

Ingredients:

- 4 bananas, peeled
- 4 cups hulled strawberries
- 4 cups spinach
- 4 cups plant-based milk

Directions:

1. Open 4 quart-size, freezer-safe bags. In each, layer in the following order: 1 banana (halved or sliced), 1 cup of strawberries, and 1 cup of spinach. Seal and place in the freezer.
2. To serve, take a frozen bag of Great Green Smoothie ingredients and transfer it to a blender. Add 1 cup of plant-based milk and blend until smooth.

Nutrition: Calories: 173 Carbohydrates: 40g Total fat: 2g Protein: 4g

39. Blueberry and Sweet Potato Smoothie

Preparation time: 5 minutes

Cooking time: 0 minutes

Servings: 1

Ingredients:

- 1/4 cup frozen blueberries
- 1/2 cup frozen sweet potato, cooked
- 1/8 teaspoon sea salt
- 1 tablespoon cacao powder
- 1 scoop of chocolate protein powder
- 1 cup almond milk

Directions:

1. Place all the ingredients in the order in a food processor or blender and then pulse for 2 to 3 minutes at high speed until smooth.
2. Pour the smoothie into a glass and then serve.

Nutrition: Calories: 150.7 Fat: 2.9 g Carbs: 27 g Protein: 7.4 g

40. Peanut Butter and Coffee Smoothie

Preparation time: 5 minutes

Cooking time: 0 minutes

Servings: 1

Ingredients:

- Small frozen banana
- 1/2 teaspoon ground turmeric
- 1 Tablespoon chia seeds
- Scoop of chocolate protein powder
- Tablespoons Peanut Butter
- Cup strong coffee, brewed

Directions:

1. Place all the ingredients in the order in a food processor or blender and then pulse for 2 to 3 minutes at high speed until smooth.
2. Pour the smoothie into a glass and then serve.

Nutrition: Calories: 189 Fat: 7 g Carbs: 24.5 g Protein: 10.3 g

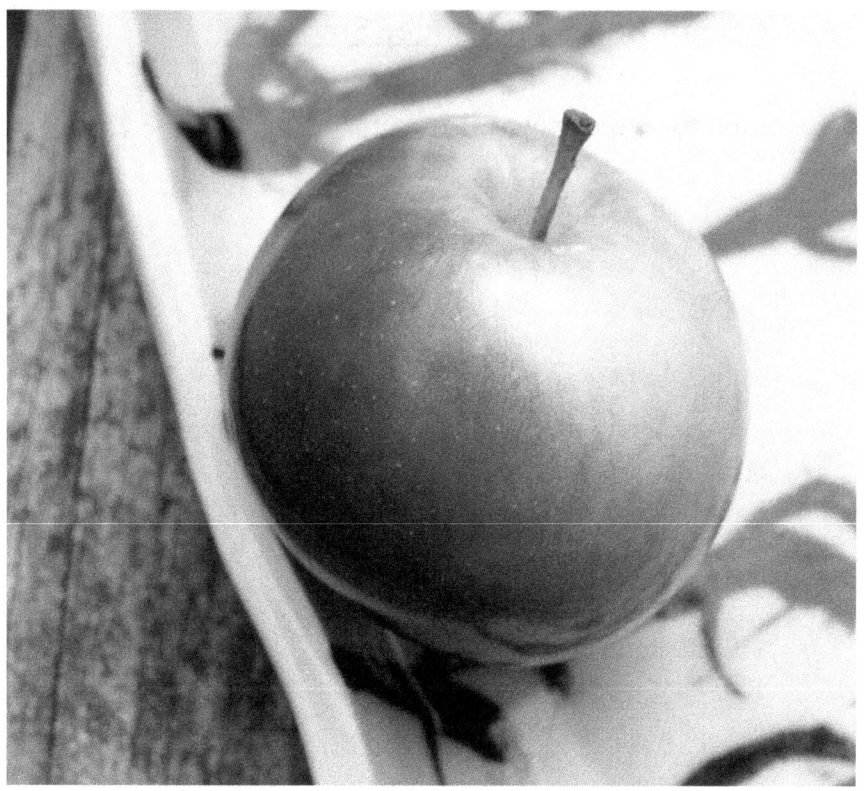

CHAPTER 8:

OTHER RECIPES

41. Lemony Romaine and Avocado Salad

Preparation Time: 15 minutes

Cooking Time: 0 minutes

Servings: 6

Ingredients:

- 1 head romaine lettuce
- ½ cup pomegranate seeds
- ¼ cup pine nuts
- ¼ cup Lemon Vinaigrette
- 2 avocados
- Freshly ground black pepper

Directions:

1. Wash your vegetables and spin-dry, then slice the leaves into bite-size pieces. Transfer the leaves to a large bowl, and toss with the pomegranate seeds, pine nuts, and half of the vinaigrette.

2. Slice the avocados in half. Remove the pit from each and slice the avocados into long thin slices. Using a large spoon, carefully scoop the slices out of the peel.

3. Arrange your avocado slices on top of the lettuce in the bowl and drizzle half of the remaining dressing over them. Carefully toss using your hands or a large metal spoon. Add the remaining dressing as needed.

4. Finish with a few sprinkles of pepper.

Nutrition: Calories: 217 Fat: 20g Carbs: 11g Protein 3g

42. Strawberry-Coconut Smoothie

Preparation Time: 10 minutes **Cooking Time:** 0 minutes

Servings: 1

Ingredients:

- Dairy-free and Vegan: Use coconut milk yogurt
- 1 cup frozen strawberries, slightly thawed
- 1 very ripe banana, sliced and frozen
- ½ cup light coconut milk
- ½ cup plain Greek yogurt
- 1 teaspoon freshly squeezed lime juice
- 1 tablespoon chia seeds (optional)
- 3 or 4 ice cubes

Directions:

1. Transfer all your ingredients to a blender and blend until smooth. If necessary, add additional coconut milk or water to thin the smoothie to your preferred consistency.

Nutrition: Calories: 278 Fat: 2g Carbs: 57g Protein: 14g

43. Aloha Mango-Pineapple Smoothie

Preparation Time: 10 minutes Cooking Time: 0 minutes

Servings: 2

Ingredients:

- 1 large navel orange, peeled and quartered
- 1 cup frozen pineapple chunks
- 1 cup frozen mango chunks
- 1 tablespoon freshly squeezed lime juice
- ½ cup plain Greek yogurt
- ½ cup milk or coconut milk
- 1 tablespoon chia seeds (optional)
- 3 or 4 ice cubes

Directions:

1. Transfer all your ingredients in a blender and blend until smooth. If necessary, add additional milk or water to thin the smoothie to your preferred consistency.

Nutrition: Calories: 158 Fat: 1g Carbs: 35g Protein: 7g

44. Lentil Soup

Preparation Time: 15 Minutes

Cooking Time: 25 Minutes

Servings: 4

Ingredients:

- 1 tbsp. Olive Oil
- 4 cups Vegetable Stock
- 1 Onion, finely chopped
- 2 Carrots, medium
- 1 cup Lentils, dried
- 1 tsp. Cumin

Directions:

1. To make this healthy soup, first, you need to heat the oil in a medium-sized skillet over medium heat.
2. Once the oil becomes hot, stir in the cumin and then the onions.
3. Sauté those for 3 minutes or until the onion is slightly transparent and cooked.

4. To this, add the carrots and toss them well.

5. Next, stir in the lentils. Mix well.

6. Now, pour in the vegetable stock and give a good stir until everything comes together.

7. As the soup mixture starts to boil, reduce the heat and allow it to simmer for 10 minutes while keeping the pan covered.

8. Turn off the heat and then transfer the mixture to a bowl.

9. Finally, blend it with an immersion blender or in a high-speed blender for 1 minute or until you get a rich, smooth mixture.

10. Serve it hot and enjoy.

Nutrition: Calories: 251 Kcal Protein: 14g Carbohydrates: 41.3g Fat: 4.1g

45. Trail Mix

Preparation Time: 10 Minutes

Cooking Time: 10 Minutes

Servings: 2

Ingredients:

- 1 cup Walnuts, raw
- 2 cups Tart Cherries, dried
- 1 cup Pumpkin Seeds, raw
- 1 cup Almonds, raw
- ½ cup Vegan Dark Chocolate
- 1 cup Cashew

Directions:

1. First, mix all the ingredients needed to make the trail mix in a large mixing bowl until combined well.
2. Store in an air-tight container.

Nutrition: Calories: 596 Kcal Protein: 17.5g Carbohydrates: 46.1g Fat: 39.5g

46. Flax Crackers

Preparation Time: 5 Minutes

Cooking Time: 60 Minutes

Servings: 4 to 6

Ingredients:

- 1 cup Flaxseeds, whole
- 2 cups Water
- ¾ cup Flaxseeds, grounded
- 1 tsp. Sea Salt
- ½ cup Chia Seeds
- 1 tsp. Black Pepper
- ½ cup Sunflower Seeds

Directions:

1. Using a large bowl, you need to put all your ingredients, then mix them well. Soak them in with water for about 10 to 15 minutes.

2. After that, transfer the mixture to a parchment paper-lined baking sheet and spread it evenly. Tip: Make sure the paper lines the edges as well.

3. Next, bake it for 60 minutes at 350 °F.

4. Once the time is up, flip the entire bar and take off the parchment paper.

5. Bake for half an hour or until it becomes crispy and browned.

6. Allow it to cool completely and then break it down.

Nutrition: Calories: 251cal Proteins: 9.2g Carbohydrates: 14.9g Fat: 16g

47. Crunchy Granola

Preparation Time: 10 Minutes

Cooking Time: 20 Minutes

Servings: 1

Ingredients:

- ½ cup Oats
- Dash of Salt
- 2 tbsp. Vegetable Oil
- 3 tbsp. Maple Syrup
- 1/3 cup Apple Cider Vinegar
- ½ cup Almonds
- 1 tsp. Cardamom, grounded

Directions:

1. Preheat the oven to 375 °F.
2. After that, mix oats, pistachios, salt, and cardamom in a large bowl.
3. Next, spoon in the vegetable oil and maple syrup to the mixture.

4. Then, transfer the mixture to a parchment-paper-lined baking sheet.

5. Bake them for 13 minutes or until the mixture is toasted. Tip: Check on them now and then. Spread it out well.

6. Return the sheet to the oven for ten minutes.

7. From your oven, remove the sheet and allow it to cool completely.

8. Serve and enjoy.

Nutrition: Calories: 763Kcal Proteins: 12.9g Carbohydrates: 64.8g Fat: 52.4g

48. Chickpea Scramble Bowl

Preparation Time: 10 Minutes

Cooking Time: 10 Minutes

Servings: Makes 2 Bowl

Ingredients:

- ¼ of 1 Onion, diced
- 15 oz. Chickpeas
- 2 Garlic cloves, minced
- ½ tsp. Turmeric
- ½ tsp. Black Pepper
- ½ tsp. Extra Virgin Olive Oil
- ½ tsp. Salt

Directions:

1. Begin by placing the chickpeas in a large bowl along with a bit of water.

2. Soak for few minutes and then mash the chickpeas lightly with a fork while leaving some of them in the whole form.

3. Next, spoon in the turmeric, pepper, and salt to the bowl. Mix well.

4. Then, heat oil in a medium-sized skillet over medium-high heat.

5. Once the oil becomes hot, stir in the onions.

6. Sauté the onions for 3 to 4 minutes or until softened.

7. Then, add the garlic and cook for 1 minute or until aromatic.

8. After that, stir in the mashed chickpeas. Cook for another 4 minutes or until thickened.

9. Serve along with micro greens. Place the greens at the bottom, followed by the scramble, and top it with cilantro or parsley.

Nutrition: Calories: 801Kcal Proteins: 41.5g Carbohydrates: 131.6g Fat: 14.7g

49. Maple Flavoured Oatmeal

Preparation Time: 5 Minutes

Cooking Time: 25 Minutes

Servings: 2

Ingredients:

- 2 tbsp. Maple Syrup
- 1 cup Oatmeal
- ½ tsp. Cinnamon
- 2 ½ cup Water
- 2/3 cup Soy Milk
- 1 tsp. Earth Balance or Vegan Butter

Directions:

1. To start with, place oatmeal and water in a medium-sized saucepan over medium-high heat.

2. Bring the mixture to a boil.

3. Next, lower the heat and cook for 13 to 15 minutes while keeping the pan covered. Tip: At this point, all the water should get absorbed by the grains.

4. Now, remove the pan from the heat and fluff this mixture with a fork.

5. Cover the pan again. Set it aside for 5 minutes.

6. Then, stir in all the remaining ingredients to the oatmeal mixture until everything comes together.

7. Serve and enjoy.

Nutrition: Calories: 411Kcal Proteins: 14.7g Carbohydrates: 73.6g Fat: 6.6g

50. Protein Pancakes

Preparation Time: 5 Minutes

Cooking Time: 10 Minutes

Servings: Makes 6 Pancakes

Ingredients:

- 1 cup All-Purpose Flour
- 2 tbsp. Maple Syrup
- ¼ cup Brown Rice Protein Powder
- ½ tsp. Sea Salt
- 1 tbsp. Baking Powder
- 1 cup Water

Directions:

1. To make these delightful protein-rich pancakes, you first need to combine the flour, sea salt, baking powder, and vegan protein powder in a large mixing bowl.

2. Spoon in the maple syrup and then later gradually add the water until you get a thick and lumpy batter.

3. Now, heat a non-stick pan over medium-high heat.

4. Then, scoop a ladle of the batter into it and cook the pancakes for 2 to 3 minutes or until bubbles form.

5. Cook each side for a further minute.

6. Serve immediately.

Nutrition: Calories: 295 Kcal Protein: 15.8g Carbohydrates: 59.9g Fat: 1.2g

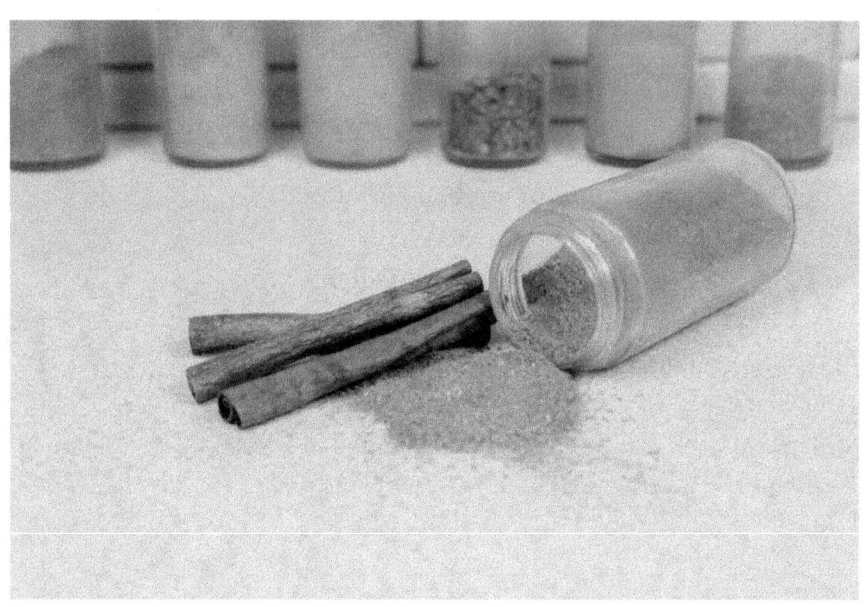

CONCLUSION

Well done! Thank you for reaching the end of this book, The Complete Vegetarian Cookbook.

Hopefully, this book has helped you understand that making vegetarian recipes and diet easier can improve your life, not only by improving your health and helping you lose weight, but also by saving you money and time.

Remember that vegetarianism is a choice, not a religion.

Be flexible when it comes to your diet and enjoy new tastes and experiences.

Don't be afraid of meat substitutes, but experiment with using them sparingly. There is no need to completely replace meat with fake meat products like tofu or processed soy-based vegetarian burgers and hot dogs. Not only are they expensive, but fake meats contain artificial ingredients that may or may not be healthy for you.

Also, if you are not used to eating a vegetarian diet, start with a few vegetarian meals and snacks during the week, and see how you feel.

You can always add more vegetarian meals to your diet later. It is better to be even slightly vegetarians than completely non-vegetarian.

The best tip I can give you about making vegetarian recipes is to experiment and have fun!

Here are some more tips to help you with your vegetarian diet:

1. Remember that vegetarianism is not a destination, it is a journey.

2. A vegetarian diet is plant-based. This means that you should try to eat more plants and less animal products. You should also be careful not to replace whole foods with their processed counterparts, such as replacing whole foods such as fruits and vegetables with fruit juice and pasta sauce.

3. Try to avoid processed food whenever possible, while still maintaining your balanced diet and nutrients that you need for your health. An easier way of doing this will be to make your own food when

possible and try to avoid packaged, pre-prepared foods at the grocery store.

4. Avoid processed food products that contain artificial ingredients, such as sweeteners, colors, and flavors.

5. Avoid highly processed meat substitutes. Remember to use meat substitutes in moderation or as an occasional treat.

6. If you choose to eat meat substitutes such as tofu, be sure to thoroughly cook it and try different ways of preparing it

7. You may need to gradually introduce your family and friends to your new eating habits. Don't expect everyone to support you or enjoy the same things you do when it comes to vegetarian recipes. As long as you are happy with your food choices, that is the most important thing – even if it means making some changes at home!

When you are having a hard time, always remember this: You can always choose to stop being a vegetarian.

You can simply start eating meat again if you are struggling with your new diet.

Remember that it is okay to be a part-time vegetarian, but if you find that you cannot maintain the lifestyle or are unhappy with your choice, it is always better to go back to eating a non-veg diet.

There is no shame in making changes to your vegetarian recipe routine if you need to, and you will not shame yourself for deciding that a strict vegetarian diet does not work for you.

I know that there are many books and choosing my book is amazing. I am thankful that you stopped and took the time to decide. You made a great decision, and I am sure that you enjoyed it.

I will be even happier if you will add some comments. Feedbacks helped by growing, and they still do. They help me to choose better content and new ideas. So, maybe your feedback can trigger an idea for my next book. Thank you again for downloading this book!

I hope you enjoyed reading my book!

www.ingramcontent.com/pod-product-compliance
Lightning Source LLC
Chambersburg PA
CBHW070936080526
44589CB00013B/1528